Sound Healing With Tuning Forks

Charles Lightwalker

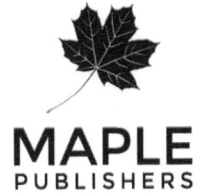

MAPLE
PUBLISHERS

Sound Healing With Tuning Forks

Author: Charles Lightwalker

Copyright © Charles Lightwalker (2023)

The right of Charles Lightwalker to be identified as author of this work has been asserted by the author in accordance with section 77 and 78 of the Copyright, Designs and Patents Act 1988.

First Published in 2024

ISBN 978-1-83538-074-1 (Paperback)

Published by:
    Maple Publishers
    Fairbourne Drive, Atterbury,
    Milton Keynes,
    MK10 9RG, UK

A CIP catalogue record for this title is available from the British Library.

All rights reserved. No part of this book may be reproduced or translated by any form or by any means, electronic or mechanical, including photocopying, recording or by any information storage and retrieval system without written permission from the author.

The views expressed in this work are solely those of the author and do not necessarily reflect the views of the publisher, and the publisher hereby disclaims any responsibility for them.

Table of Contents

Forward	4
Introduction	6
Funing Forks	8
Tuning Forks and Healing	10
How to Use Tuning Forks	14
Using Tuning Forks With The chakra System	18
Other Uses For Tuning Forks	40
Reflex Points	43
Tuning the Organs	47
Body Tuning	53
Aterthoughts	
Articles on Tuning Forks	

Forward to Revised Edition 2023

The time has come to release again this manual/book on sound healing with tuning forks, that I wrote in 2005, and used as a manual with the tuning fork classes I was teaching at that time in my life. I was also working with various other sound healers through the tuning fork research alliance, as we were experiencing the use of tuning forks with other healing modalities and working with research scientists to discover the vibrational frequencies that could be used on specific ailments, illnesses, and problems that were occurring to the human form, and on how to use tuning forks on the treatment of animals. The research is continuing and I have no doubt that the art of healing using tuning forks will expand the health of many and contribute to the knowledge of complimentary care worldwide. May this book contribute to the expanding of knowledge in the sound healing arts.   Charles- summer 2023-Scotland

Introduction

TUNING FORK PROCESSES
COMMON TERMS USED

- AcuTuning - A process where tuning forks are used to tune the meridian points found in standard acupuncture processes.
- Angel Armour - A process to release stress and tension from the muscle and areas of the body (found in AcuTuning 2 Manual).
- Angel - A Messenger of God or the Divine Presence in all things.
- Chakra - Energy Centers in the body.
- Frequency - The number of repetitions per unit time of a complete wave.
- Grace - This is the life giving energy found in all things.
- Hertz - Measurements of cycles in hundreds.
- HZ - This means hertz.
- Oil - This is referring to the sacred angelic essential oils. These are a blend of essential oils that are blessed and laid to rest to increase their frequencies. For more information see oil information sheet or the Sacred Angelic Oils Manual.
- Prongs - The two ends of the fork, shaped like a U, which vibrate.
- Reflex - The process of pointing the prongs at an area of the body or by placing it on one area of the body to affect another; such as foot reflexology.
- Stem - This is the handle of the tuning fork.
- Tune - Putting an area back into proper frequency. Example: tuning a guitar.
- Tuning Fork Practitioner- a certified tuning fork healer
- TFRA- Tuning Fork Research Alliance

- Tuning Fork Therapist- a term used by some tuning fork practitioners
- Vibration - This is what you feel when the tuning fork is vibrating or moving back and forth.
- Wash - This is where you point the prongs of the tuning fork at the area you are working on.
- Wave - A disturbance or osculation propagated from point to point by mathematical specifications of its amplitude.
- Wave Form - Is the mechanic representation of a wave.

TUNING FORKS

Tuning forks are very precise instruments for producing sounds at a given frequency. They are made out of two basic materials, stainless steel, and aluminum. Aluminum alloy tuning forks are usually used in health and healing applications and emit a tone that is more pure, vibrant, and longer lasting than stainless steel. You are also able to produce overtones and harmonics with aluminum forks that cannot be produced with stainless steel forks. Stainless steel tuning forks are capable of producing only one tone.

The only advantage to stainless steel is that the material is harder than aluminum. Accordingly, more care and gentle handling needs to be given to aluminum tuning forks. It is important to note that regardless of the material being used, all tuning forks are slightly affected by temperature and elevation above sea level. Tuning forks can be purchased with weighted or unweighted ends.

Weighted ends produce a stronger vibration with a louder overall sound that lasts longer and also allows you to better feel the vibration when the stem end is placed on the body. Weighted tuning forks weigh considerably more than standard tuning forks and can be tiring to hold for long periods of time. They also cost considerably more than the standard tuning fork. Unweighted tuning forks are therefore more economical and practical to use for healing purposes.

There are a wide variety of tuning forks available for all types of applications. If there's a frequency, there's a tuning fork ...or two. Tuning forks are all designed around frequencies and the mathematical formulas that determine progressions of frequencies. Some fork sets are based around the mathematics of the solar system, others on the individual planets or their orbits, some on each individual organ of the body as well as individual types of body cells and DNA nucleotides. Tuning forks can be found that supposedly resonate to mineral nutrients, elements, dimensions, the sun, the moon, and a wide range of other non-physical phenomena such as astral projection. Each frequency has a purpose. Do they work? One would have to look for and at results to make this determination or perhaps accept the fact that sometimes things work for reasons that cannot be quantitatively or qualitatively measured. Perhaps it is a matter of faith and intention.

This manual will focus on the use of a standard set of Pythagorean tuning forks and includes several methods for balancing and aligning the Chakras. A variety of tuning forks having special uses will also be presented. Solfeggio Scale tuning forks will also be introduced along with some techniques for their use. Finally, the use of tuning forks in other healing modalities will be presented.

Tuning Forks and Healing

The human body functions harmonically. The frequencies of breathing, blood circulation, the pulse, and all the activities associated with them are intended to function in harmonic balance. Since sound affects us at both the conscious and unconscious levels it has the effect of counterbalancing the physical and emotional states of the body and the mind. By using sound, the internal and external can be brought back into harmony and flexibility. Tuning forks create a resonance throughout our mind, body, emotions, and etheric body. As such, they are powerful tools to facilitate balancing and healing.

A tuning fork, when struck, produces a single sound or note with harmonics and overtones of that note. Strike two tuning forks together and two vibrational frequencies are created. The brain however, hears more than just the two frequencies. It also hears a third frequency derived from the difference between the two forks. So in actuality the brain hears three vibrational frequencies from just the two forks. It follows then, that when multiple forks are used, many harmonics, overtones, and frequencies are experienced. Think of it as bathing in sound.

When tuning forks are used as a tool for healing, the vibrational frequency coupled with the intent can cause a healing effect to occur. The intention for healing to occur must be considered before beginning a session using tuning forks. During a healing session it is not uncommon for others to experience the intention behind the sound. The intention 'rides along' with the sound wave. It is equally important that the client be receptive to the sound and its accompanying intention. This can be accomplished by making sure the recipient is expecting to hear the tones and that he or she is in a relaxed state. It is important to remember that in all aspects of the healing arts the relationship and communication between the practitioner and the client is very important.

A healthy body is in perfect harmonic balance. When the body is out of balance tuning forks can be used to bring about major, positive shifts in the energy patterns within and surrounding the human body. The frequencies generated by the forks act to dissolve negative energy in the aura and chakras. Sound vibration and intent can clear out energy blocks quickly and effectively. During tuning fork therapy, a beneficial process of resonance occurs. As the correct frequency is focused on various parts of the body, new patterns of balance are laid down that essentially can erase old patterns caused by the negative resonance of ill health. If a part of the body is out of balance it will energetically resonate `out of tune'. By applying the correct frequency a resonance is created that entrains the part that is out of balance

back to its correct frequency. The body or body area will only take in and absorb whatever vibrations are needed so sound therapy is a very safe form of therapy to use, even on children. Sound has other effects at conscious and unconscious levels. Sound may often evoke emotional responses and can counterbalance negative emotional states of the body and mind.

Sound can also:

- Energize the body
- Soothe and balance the nervous system
- Lift the spirit
- Promote an almost instantaneous deep state of relaxation
- Promote a meditative state
- Improve mental clarity
- Enhance brain functioning
- Increase mental concentration
- 'Center' the body
- Enhance massage, meditation, Reiki, and acupressure
- Balance and integrate both sides of the brain

- Balance and realign the chakras
- Clear and charge the aura
- Clear and raise the vibrational frequency of a room
- Be used on all acupuncture points and meridians

How To Use Tuning Forks

Tuning forks are very easy to use and take very little practice, without effort or damaging them. It is advisable to practice the various ways to activate tuning forks so that you become comfortable in their use. Remember that these are precision instruments and can be damaged if carelessly used or mistreated.

The tuning fork is generally held one of two ways. The 'stem' end is held very gently, a bit loosely, between the fingers at the bottom of the fork. Be sure not to be too close to the body of the tuning fork. If your fingers or hand comes in contact with the vibrating body of the tuning fork the vibrations will stop. The tuning fork can also be placed in the palm of the hand between the thumb and the index finger. When used in contact with the practitioner's palm it is said the vibrations also act as a carrier for channeling the healing energy of the practitioner into the fork, through the fork, and out the fork ends. Be sure not to touch or hang on to the tines of the tuning fork as that will dampen or stop the vibration.

Striking it against a hard rubber object such as a hockey puck, rubber dog bone, or a rubber mallet activates the fork. You can also activate it by striking it against your knee or on the palm of your hand. This will produce a somewhat softer sound. Striking the fork gently on your kneecap can produce a loud sound. You do not need to use a lot of force. A quick flicking motion is all that is required. If a louder sound is desired strike the tuning fork twice in succession against the hard rubber object or gently tap two tuning forks against each other being careful not to nick the edges. If the tuning fork is weighted, the weighted end can be quickly pinched together and released or hit against the heel of the palm of the opposite hand. Do not strike a weighted tuning fork so forcefully that the ends knock together.

It is wise to avoid striking two tuning forks together. If the edges are chipped or dinged the frequency will be altered.

Rarely is this admonition violated but when forks must be struck together it should be done very gently and never on the edges.

If essential oils are used and your tuning forks have painted stems make sure to carefully clean off any oil that might get on them. This will ensure that the paint does not degrade or come off.

Taking care of the tuning forks

The use of Tuning Forks is on the rise within the healing profession. There are a few things to know about tuning forks and their use to have them last you a very long time.

The first is their care. Use a soft rubber object to strike them on. A hockey puck is what we have found to work the best. Also a rubber dog bone works well. Never strike them on anything hard like a table or for that matter hitting them together. This damages the forks and changes their frequencies. And it is the frequencies that are doing the work anyway. Also it is not necessary to hit the fork very hard at all. If you hit it to hard you can bend the fork or damage it and change the frequency. Just lightly tap the fork, usually from the wrist, on the hockey puck. This will cause it to lightly vibrate and you may or may not hear the tone loudly. Some of the forks are very high frequencies and they are not very loud. So louder is not better.

Second is storage. It is best to store them in the bags they came with. This is so they do not clank together or if they do get dropped they have some cushion to fall on. We have a box we carry all of our forks in. You want to make sure that there is a layer of bubble wrap between the layers of forks so that the forks do not clang together in the box as well.

Third is the color on the forks. This can come off. Be careful when using your forks and the oils together. Also if the forks clang together it can result in chipping and peeling of the paint. Avoid striking the handles together to keep the handles the beautiful colors that they are. Due to normal wear and tear on the forks during use the paint may peel. There are a few things that can be done to have the color last longer; wash your hands after handling essential oils and before using the forks, do not bang the forks together, avoid hitting the painted end on anything which can result in chipping, If oil does get on the handle of the forks wipe it off with soap and water, then allow to air dry. Also when using the frequencies for healing, know that no harm can come from applying them to a different area than called for. The frequency will not cause anything to go wrong or cause any damage. It will simply pass through the body unchanged.

Using Tuning Forks with the Chakra System

An assumption is being made that anyone using this manual already possesses an understanding of the Chakra System. A more in-depth presentation on the glands and various states of physical dysfunction associated with each chakra is beyond the scope of this manual. Many fine books are in circulation that contains in-depth presentations of each chakra.

The chakras, the body's energy centers, can be thought of as being a series of steps or lessons one must learn as they ascend from the physical level to the Divine level. Carolyn Myss, in her book "Anatomy of the Spirit", says that each chakra is the center for a particular power. These powers ascend from the densest physical power to the most spiritual power. She states that these powers seem to match the challenges we face in our lives. Each chakra is also associated with various glands and functions of the body.

The standard set of tuning forks can be used in many ways when the characteristics, glands, and powers of each chakra are considered. They may be used to enhance meditation on each chakra, clear out old patterns, release blockages, clear out congestion, physical dysfunctions, and raise our vibratory level to help our efforts to work through or with any of the challenges the chakras represent.

Following are just a few of the many characteristics, issues, emotions, mental areas, and glands in which tuning forks might be of value. The more one knows about the positive and negative attributes or characteristics of the chakra system, the more versatile the tuning forks become.

The Eleven-Chakra System
A Brief Outline by Sherry Fields

The human body contains hundreds of locations where there is focused and concentrated energy. There are, however, twelve major energy centers, commonly referred to as "chakras." Chakra is a Sanskrit word, which means, "wheel." The chakras are similar to wheels in that they are spinning vortexes of energy. They are centers of force located within our etheric body, through which we receive, transmit, and process life energies.

Eastern philosophy has taught a system based on seven chakras for thousands of years and is the basis for spiritual growth in many cultures. Today the angelic realms are teaching a Twelve Chakra system based on lost and forgotten information that will serve as tools to assist humanity in its spiritual journey.

Each chakra in the body is recognized as a focal point for life-force relating to spiritual, physical, emotional, and mental energies. The chakras are the network through which the mind, body, and spirit interact as one holistic system. These major chakras correspond to specific aspects of our consciousness and have their own individual characteristics and functions. Most have a corresponding relationship to one of the various glands of the body's endocrine system, as well as to colors of the rainbow spectrum.

The main purpose in working with and understanding the chakras is to create integration and wholeness within ourselves. In this way we bring the various aspects of our consciousness from the physical to the spiritual, into a harmonious relationship. Ultimately, we begin to recognize that the various aspects of ourselves all work together, and that each aspect is as much a part of the whole as the others. We must be able to acknowledge, integrate, and accept all levels of our being.

To help us in the process of our unfolding it is most important to understand that the chakras are doorways for our consciousness. They are the doorways through which emotional, mental, and spiritual force flow into physical _expression. They are openings through which our attitudes and belief systems enter into and create our mind/ body structure. The energy created from our emotional and mental attitudes runs though the chakras and is distributed to our cells, tissues and organs. Realizing this brings tremendous insight into how we ourselves affect our bodies, minds, and circumstances for better or for worse. To understand the chakras and their relationship to our consciousness is to better understand ourselves. Understanding ourselves will enable us to make our choices and decisions from a place of balance and awareness, rather than being blindly influenced by forces we do not understand.

This outline is a brief description only. For more comprehensive information on the first seven chakras please refer to the many books on the subject. Two good ones are "The Energy of Anatomy" by Carolyn Myss and "The Wheels of Life" by Anodea Judith.

FIRST CHAKRA: ROOT or BASE CHAKRA

Location: Base of the spine (coccyx)
Color: Red (secondary color is black)
Element: Earth
Functions: Gives vitality to the physical body. Life-force survival, self-preservation, instincts survival. Relationship to our tribe, our community, and our family.
Glands /organs: Adrenals, kidneys, spinal column, leg bones.
Gems /minerals: Ruby, garnet, bloodstone, red jasper, black tourmaline, obsidian, and smoky quartz.
Foods: Proteins, Red fruits and vegetables.
Associated aromas: Cedar, Clove
Sensory function: Smell
Qualities /lessons: Matters relating to the material world, success. The physical body, mastery of the body. Grounding, individuality, stability, security, stillness, health, courage, and patience.
Negative qualities: Self-centered, insecurity, violence, greed, and anger.

SECOND CHAKRA: SPLEEN CHAKRA (Sacral Plexus)

Location: Lower abdomen to navel area
Color: Orange
Element: Water
Functions: Procreation, assimilation of food, physical force and vitality, sexuality.
Glands /organs: Ovaries, testicles, prostrate gland, genitals, spleen, womb, and bladder.
Gems /Minerals: Carnelian, coral, gold calcite, amber, citrine, gold topaz, and peach aventurine.
Foods: Liquids: Orange fruits and vegetables.
Associated aromas: Ylang/Ylang, Sandalwood
Sensory function: Taste
Qualities/lessons: Giving & receiving emotions, desire, pleasure, sexual /passionate love, change, movement, assimilation of new ideas. Health, family tolerance, and surrender. Working harmoniously and creatively with others.
Negative qualities: Overindulgence in food or sex, sexual difficulties, confusion, purposelessness, jealousy, envy, desire to possess, emotionalism.

THIRD CHAKRA: SOLAR PLEXUS

Location: Below the breastbone and behind the stomach.
Color: Golden Yellow.
Element: Fire
Functions: It is the center of personal power, ambition, intellect, astral force, desire, and emotions based on intellect and touch.
Glands/organs: Pancreas, liver, digestive tract, stomach, Liver, spleen, gall bladder, autonomic nervous system.
Gems/minerals: Tiger's Eye, Amber, Yellow Topaz, and Citrine.
Foods: Complex Carbohydrates, and Grains.
Associated aromas: Lavender, Rosemary, and Bergamot.
Sensor- function: Sight.
Qualities/lessons: Transforming. Shaping, Purifying, Shaping of Being, Mental Energy.
Negative qualities: Perfectionism, control over self versus others, self-critical thoughts, frustration, anxiety.

FOURTH CHAKRA: HEART CHAKRA

Location: Center of chest, at level of heart.
Color: Green (secondary color is pink).
Element: Air.
Functions: It is the center, which vitalizes the heart, thymus, circulatory system, blood, cellular structure, and involuntary muscles.
Glands/organs: Heart, ribs, chest cavity, lower lungs, and blood, circulatory system, skin, hands, and thymus.
Gems/minerals: Kunzite, emerald, green jade, rose quartz, and pink tourmaline.
Foods: Green vegetables, dark leafy greens.
Associated aromas: Rose oil.
Sensory function: Touch.
Qualities/lessons: The center of compassion, love, group consciousness, and spirituality associated with "oneness" with "all that is." It provides for desegregation between the loving energy of the heart and the analytical energy of the intellect. God connection. Able to give and receive. Open to change and new ideas. Coping with loss. Balance.
Negative qualities: Self-abandonment, fear, sadness, anger, resentment, jealousy, and hostility.

FIFTH CHAKRA: THROAT CHAKRA

Location: Neck, throat area above collarbone.
Color: Blue
Element: The higher _expression of all signs.
Functions: Communication center, acting to provide the energy for, and the understanding of, both verbal and mental communications.
Glands/Organs: Thyroid gland, throat and jaw areas, alimentary canal, lungs, vocal cords, and the breath.
Gems/minerals: Aquamarine, Turquoise, Chalcedony, Chrysocolla.
Foods: Fruit.
Associated aromas: Sage, eucalyptus.
Sensory function: Hearing.
Qualities/lessons: The gateway to the Higher Consciousness and the gateway through which the emotions contained on the heart must pass to become balanced and harmonized. Open, clear communication of feelings and thoughts. Creativity, speaking up, releasing, and healing.
Negative qualities: Uptight, low self-esteem, low self-confidence, hostility, anger, and resentment.

SIXTH CHAKR.A: THIRD EYE (BROW CHAKRA)

Location: Between and about one finger-breadth above the eyebrows.
Color: Indigo
Element: The higher _expression of all signs.
Functions: The center of psychic power, higher intuition, the energies of the spirit, Magnetic forces, and light. Clairvoyance, healing addictions. Central Nervous system.
Gems/minerals: Lapis lazuli, indigo, sapphire, sodalite.
Foods: Chlorophyll, breath, and air.
Associated aromas: Mint, jasmine.
Sensory function: all, inclusive ESP.
Qualities/lessons: Higher consciousness, emotional and spiritual love center, Spiritual inner sight, clairvoyance. When balanced, the mind (right hemisphere) and brain (left hemisphere) function in a Unified field. Insight ensues and its practical application becomes a daily occurrence. It also assists in the purification of negative tendencies and in the elimination of selfish attitudes.
Negative qualities: Worry, hysteria, stress, fear, shock, irritation, depression, headaches, speech and weight problems.

SEVENTH CHAKRA: CROWN CHAKRA

Location: Crown of head.
Color: Violet.
Element: The higher _expression of all elements.
Function: The center of spirituality, enlightenment, dynamic thought and energy. It is the center that vitalizes the cerebrum, the right eye, and the pineal gland.
Glands/organs: Pineal gland, cerebrum.
Gems/minerals: Amethyst, quartz crystal.
Foods: Sun, juice, fasting.
Associated aromas: Galbanum, lotus.
Sensory function: None
Qualities/lessons: It allows for the inward flow of wisdom from the ethers and brings the gift of cosmic consciousness. When stimulated and clear, it enables one to see the truth concerning illusory ideals, materialistic pursuits, self-limiting concepts, pride, and vanity; it further allows one to experience continuous self-awareness and conscious detachment from personal emotions, compassion, seeing self in others, peacefulness, oneness.
Negative qualities: Confusion, anxiety, stress.
Additional Chakras as described by Metatron

EIGHTH CHAKRA - INFRA RED – OMEGA

Location: Midway between the root chakra and the knees
Color: Infrared, a combination of red and blue
Function: An energy transference chakra. It takes in energy from the world and other people, plants and animals and operates like a step-down or step-up transformer. Seeing the whole body and the Chakras as an integrated energy system, the Omega transfers energy from outside the body to inside increasing or decreasing it as necessary to stimulate energy flow and release blocks.
Qualities/lessons: It is also like a two-way valve, we can use the Omega to release stored/stagnant Chi or energy, or for clearing a block/learning the lesson. Used to release also when we ask the angels/spirit to assist us to transmute negative thoughts and belief systems, past words, actions or deeds.
Negative qualities: Inactivity/sloth, emotionalism - empathic abilities run riot, getting into other people's stuff and not focusing on self growth.

NINTH CHAKRA - ULTRA VIOLET – ALPHA

Location: Between 12 and 18 inches out from the top of the head.
Color: Ultra Violet - blue and violet
Function: This chakra is the access to information about Karma, lessons, our learning abilities, doorways to dimensions and times as well as the Akashic records. When we access past life information it is through this chakra. Occasionally we can access this information in the dream state, when there is important information to be communicated to us. Often spirit/angels will use this tool to get our attention. The dream state many times expresses ideas in symbols and it is our job to interpret the symbols presented. We can of course gain confirmation of our interpretation through meditation. But first the idea or lesson must be accessed.
Qualities/lessons: Innate knowledge of the law of Karma, other dimensions and Akashic records, past life interpretation
Negative qualities: Too much reliance on outside guidance, looses communication with the higher self within.

TENTH CHAKRA - SILVER – TERRA

Location: Midway between the knees and the feet.
Color: Silver
Function: The Grounding Chakra, a receptive energy with a positive flow containing the elements of wind, earth, water and fire. It is the anchor to the physical world. We are spiritual beings having a physical experience. We need to stay balanced, emotionally, mentally, physically and spiritually.
Equally the chakras must be balanced. We are not just to work on the spiritual or upper chakras, but all of them equally. We are here in the physical for a purpose to learn and grow through the experience. It is through the Terra Chakra that we ground and connect to the earth (Gaia). This is where our sense of knowing 'nature' develops and understanding the naturalness of the cycles of life. Birth, growth then death. It is repeated everywhere in nature, in the plant life, the animal life, the mineral life even in the cosmos.
Qualities/lessons: Keeping balance here helps us to stay grounded and understand the nature of our life, the cycles and the patterns within it. It allows us to develop our natural knowing.
Negative qualities: In the unbalanced, ungrounded state we develop fears about the cycles of life, loose connection with our spiritual knowing.

ELEVENTH CHAKRA - GOLD – ANGELIC

Location: Between 18 and 24 inches out from the top of our head
Color: Gold
Function: The angelic chakra contains the programming of the soul for this lifetime and the history of the soul. It is through our connection and understanding of this chakra that we gain or

affect our own healings, insights, learn our lessons, understand the soul contracts and begin to understand our life purpose.

Qualities/lessons: As we continue to evolve as physical/spiritual beings our understanding of this chakra is strengthened. We can begin to see (re-remember) the goals we came into this life to achieve. As we grow in understanding we can endeavor to achieve those goals by living our life in the flow of its purpose instead of against it.

Negative Qualities: None, communication from the angelic realm cannot be negative.

Chakra Balancing

Tuning forks are an effective and fast way to balance the Chakra system. The Chakras can be balanced using a standard set of seven or eight Pythagorean tuning forks, or a set of seven Solfeggio tuning forks. Instructions will also be given for using a set of seven tuning forks to balance a system of twelve chakras.

For the procedures to follow we will use a standard set of seven Pythagorean tuning forks. These forks span a tonal range from C at 256 Hz to B at 481 Hz. Some sets will include an eighth fork, which makes a full octave of sound, but this isn't required for balancing the seven chakras.

If a chakra is out of balance in any way, closed down, too small, not circular in spin, or out to the side, exposure to the tones will cause it to immediately realign, balance, and open up. It may take several balancing sessions to `train' an out of balance chakra to hold or remain in a balanced position. In a sense, the chakra must `forget' the frequency of being out of balance and `learn' the new and correct frequency. Of course any personal or health issues that might be the source of imbalance must be addressed.

To begin all procedures the tuning forks will be activated as described earlier and either held over the chakra, circled over the chakra, or have the stem end placed on the chakra. Let your intuition guide you as to what is required. Several methods of chakra balancing will be presented.

Balancing and Opening the Chakras

This method balances all seven of the chakras. Start with the C and G tuning forks to relax the client. This is the Body Tuning process presented earlier in the manual.

If you have the Shekinah and Michael tuning forks from Angel Gate Creations you can use the Shekinah tuning fork to ground the client and the Michael fork to call in Spirit. Additional information on these tuning forks is located in the section titled Angel Forks.

Tone the C tuning fork and begin to balance the system starting at the root chakra and proceed up through the 7th or Crown chakra.

Once activated keep the tuning fork several inches above the chakra, about 6 to 8 inches will do. It is not necessary to be any closer. Point the ends of the tuning fork down and over the chakra. You may also move the tuning fork around the chakra in a clockwise motion to vibrationally encourage the chakra to open further. Hold the tuning fork in this position for approximately 20 to 30 seconds or until you can no longer hear or feel the vibration.

If your set has an eighth tuning fork you may use it for the Transpersonal chakra. You may then also use the C and G forks again, or the Creation fork, to sweep the body from head to toe or circle the body to balance and seal the etheric fields.

When using the tuning forks to balance your own chakras you might try visualizing the colors of each chakra as you tune them. Visualize a ball of color at the location of the chakra and as you hear the sound, draw it into the ball of color.

Chakra Connecting

This method of balancing the chakras can be done using the techniques of presented in Chakra Balancing.

As they are tuned and balanced each chakra will be linked with the one directly above it. Start at the root chakra and balance it. Before you finish with this chakra slowly sweep the energy up to the sacral chakra, thus making an energy link from the root chakra to the sacral. Now, proceed on to tune the sacral chakra and finish with a sweep up to the solar plexus. Balance the remaining chakras in this manner. As you finish with the crown chakra sweep the energy around the body's auric field from top to bottom three times.

Balancing the Chakras with a Heart Link

This method will involve keeping a link between the heart and each of the seven chakras as they are balanced. Use any of the Chakra Balancing techniques. The practitioner will hold their right hand over or lightly touching the heart chakra while balancing each chakra with the tuning forks held in the left hand. The frequency of the tuning forks will also travel directly to the chakras through the body of the practitioner, through the heart, and out of their right hand down to the heart of the client. The healing energy the practitioner brings to the session will also pass to the client along with the tuning fork vibrations. At the heart chakra hold the tuning fork over the hand that is holding position over or on the heart.

To avoid having crossed arms it will be necessary to switch sides of the table to complete the remaining chakras from the Throat to the Crown.

Balancing the Chakras to the Heart

This variation of chakra balancing will balance the lower chakras as in Chakra Linking except that all chakras will balance to the Heart and not beyond. The lower chakras will balance up to the Heart and the upper chakras will balance down to the Heart.

Balance the Root chakra and sweep the vibration up to the Heart. Next balance the Sacral chakra and sweep the vibration up to the Heart as well. Repeat with the Solar Plexus chakra. The upper chakras will balance and sweep down to the Heart chakra in the same manner the lower chakras were balanced. The Heart chakra will be balanced last.

One way to complete this session is to hold all of the tuning forks except the Heart tuning fork in the left hand and very gently activate them by striking them with the Heart fork in order from Root to Crown. Be very careful not to strike the tuning forks too hard or the tines may get dinged or chipped. Do not strike the tuning forks directly on their edges. Wash over the entire body with the tuning forks, starting at the feet and coming back to end at the Heart chakra. The sound of all the tuning forks activated at once is very harmonious and soothing to the client.

Chakra Readings

All sorts of energies and issues may be found in the chakras. The chakras are funnel shaped and have four wheels or rings within them that correspond to the physical, emotional, mental and spiritual bodies. The innermost rings in this spiraling energy are smaller than the outside rings. Healthy rings spin clockwise in the northern hemisphere (opposite in the southern hemisphere). The chakras in front of the person represent the conscious and the chakras in back of the person represent the unconscious. There is a chakra bridge in between. Always read and assist in clearing the front chakras first.

If any chakras are spinning counter clockwise (in NH), start the clearing there. Some reasons for a counter clockwise spin are:
1. A physical whack
2. A very intrusive cord
3. Clingy control energy
4. Lots of foreign energy with a charge on it.
5. Chakra is releasing something.

You can use a pendulum to ask which direction a chakra is rotating. With practice you can tell by feeling with your hand or just trust your knowing.

Reading and Clearing the Chakras:

1. Put a picture of the chakra on your screen. Throw purple at it and see if it sticks anywhere. Run your hand over the screen to feel for cords and foreign energy. Listen for guidance, pay attention to the first thought that enters your mind. Look at the front first and then the back.
2. Look for pain, perfect pictures, whacks, other people, belief systems, thought forms, cords, and contracts.
3. Ask the person's higher self what is appropriate to assist in clearing at this time. Person may not be ready to let go of some things as they are still serving them in some way.
4. Decording - Do not take out cords the person may still be dependent on or good cords (i.e. between the heart chakras of lovers, between mothers and young children). There may be homework for the person to do if there is a dependent cord. The person may go into shock or terror if it is removed prematurely. If the cord is to be removed, take it out with a rose. If it won't stay out, there is probably a contract that needs to be cleared attached to the cord.

5. To clear contracts have the client mentally write it on a piece of paper, rip it up and violet flame it. To clear beliefs and perfect pictures, have the client visualize a snap shot of the belief, stamp cancel all over it and violet flame it.
6. Erase pain, reweave whacks with golden filaments.
7. Other people - ask why person has let someone else into their chakra; there may be a contract or belief. Once reason is cleared, have client push a picture of the person outside of their aura with their breath and blow them up in a rose.

Preparing to Do a Reading

1. Put down a grounding cord. Pull your aura into 18 to 24 inches from your body.
2. Contact and acknowledge your higher self. Ask for assistance with the reading and healing.
3. Put fresh roses around your aura.
4. Adjust your first, second and third chakras.
a. Adjust the first and second chakras to ten percent open. This helps you to be in a healthy state of detachment and not take on other people's emotions. It allows your clairsentience to be more open and feel the energies.
b. Adjust your third chakra to 70 percent open for women and 50 percent open for men. This allows you to have more confidence in yourself and the information you are receiving.
5. Place a large neutralizing Reading and Healing Rose with a grounding cord between your aura and the client's aura with the intent that it will take on cords, energies etc. that are clearing from the other instead of getting into your space.
6. Place a Matching Picture Rose between your and their auras. When you have a matching issue it will pull energy out of the energy field, acting like a photocopier, healing you as well.
   a. Optional - Place a matching picture rose at each chakra.
7. Observe the color of their Crown Loop on your screen and match yours one shade (frequency) lighter. You may set your crown loop color by intention. This keeps you from drawing their energy into your aura.
8. Put up your "TV" reading screen between your aura and the reading and healing rose. Option- connect two grounding cords to the screen.
9. If someone is blocking the screen or trying to get into your space, hook them up to the Supreme Being and have them pulled out of your space.

10. Visualize a golden sun above your head and bring the light down through your crown chakra through the pineal gland, to the throat, then down both arms ending in the palms of your hands. Run the energy across the screen to clear it.

11. Ask the client to say their name three times and touch the screen to feel it as they are saying it. This will give you a sense of their energy signature.

a. If their current name is not the same as their birth name, have them say their birth name twice and their current name twice.

b. Option: ground them on the screen.

12. Anchor your crown loop to the four corners of the room. This helps you own the space during the reading.

13. Tune into their being, in and out of their body. Say hello to their Higher Self and ask permission to do the reading. (Sometimes they say no.)

Ending a Reading
Making Separations:

1. Blow the matching picture rose.
2. Put the client's face in a rose and run it through your aura to pick up any energy that may have stuck to you.
3. Blow the healing rose.
4. Visualize a golden ring with a piece missing and ask that anything that has not been completed in the reading be completed. Fill in the missing space with golden light. Then blow the ring up in a rose.
5. Tear and burn the contract between you and the other person. "My agreement to do this reading is now complete in the physical and other realms /realities".
6. Do five physical separations. Look at the person and identify five things about them that is not you. That is them, it is not me.
7. Affirm "My energy will run in perfect order to take care of me. My energy will run in a way that is in affinity with me."
8. Allow the chakras to come back to normal operating percentages. Put any second chakra stuff in a second chakra rose and blow it up.

Other Uses for Tuning Forks

Once activated the tuning fork can be used in several different ways depending on the type of treatment being given or its intended use. To determine which tuning fork to use, consider the intention behind the action. To raise the vibratory level before a healing session, a class, or meditation, choose a fork with a high frequency, such as the tuning fork that vibrates to the note of B. If the intention is to ground an individual or a room, use a tuning fork of a lower frequency such as the tuning fork for the note C. The Solfeggio tuning forks are an excellent choice for use in healing when intention is being considered but the Pythagorean tuning forks are equally useful.

Here are some other ways to use tuning forks:

1. The tines (ends) can be pointed at the area to be treated allowing the vibration to focus onto or into the specific part of the body, organ, energy block, or area of discomfort or pain.
2. Sound energy from the ends of the tuning fork can be focused directly into the center of a chakra or meridian point. Keep several inches between the fork and the client.
3. The energy can be spiraled into and around a chakra to balance and gently open the chakra even further.
4. The tuning fork can be 'washed' over a large area, bathing the area in vibration. To enhance spiritual states try using one or more of the tuning forks that have a high frequency. Useful in enhancing your personal space.
5. The fork can be waved around the body to clear, charge, balance, or clean the auric field. You would use a tuning fork with a high vibration.

6. Activate more than one fork and stroke the chakras, the body's energy field, meridian lines, or the entire body.
7. Use two tuning forks, such as the C and G fork, to balance the body, left / right, front / back or top / bottom.
8. The stem end can be placed directly onto an area to send the vibrations into the tissues, bones, joints, muscles, energy block, acupuncture points, acupressure points, energy tines, chakras, etc.
9. Tuning forks can be used with crystals. One example would be to direct a crystal point, one whose other end is flat, towards a chakra, activate a tuning fork and touch the stem end of the tuning fork to the flat end of the crystal. The tuning fork vibration will be enhanced as it passes through the crystal. If you use crystals or stones in your chakra or Reiki sessions you can charge them using the tuning fork that corresponds to the chakra. Activate the tuning fork, point it, move it around, or touch the stem end to the crystal or stone.
10. Use the stem end to charge objects such as, crystals, stones, water, etc. Activate the tuning fork and place the stem end gently against the object. Water can be charged by actually gently touching the surface of the water with the tines of an activated tuning fork two or three times.
11. Charge your food by sweeping over it with a tuning fork. Perhaps a good choice would be a tuning fork that has an attribute or characteristic of gratitude or love. The tuning fork for the heart chakra, the note F, would be a good choice.
12. Tuning forks can be used to set the vibrational level of a room prior to or after an event. Use a high vibration tuning fork to bring in Spirit. Use a low vibration tuning fork to ground the room.
13. Tuning forks can be used in a wide variety of other healing uses such as Reiki, hypnotherapy, massage, reflexology, yoga, meditation, color therapy, psychotherapy, pain management, and sports rehabilitation.

14. In any healing application, for example Reiki, tuning forks can be used to set the vibrational level of the room, ground the client, call in higher vibrations, and tune the client for the session (see Body Tuning and Om fork). The Reiki symbols can also be drawn in the air using a tuning fork such as the Om, Creation, or any of a high vibration.
15. You can learn to use your voice to resonate with the sound of a tuning fork. Hum with the sound of the tuning fork and later use your mind to produce the sound. By practicing this you can then carry the sound of the frequencies internally and resonate with any fork at any time. The Om fork might be a good tuning fork to learn to hum to. This process is called Toning and was developed by John Beaulieu, N. D. founder of The BioSonic Academy.

Remember, the more you use and experiment with tuning forks the more uses you will discover for them. It is helpful to keep a log of how you use your tuning forks along with a notation of the effect or results from each use. Keep in mind that not all clients will respond in the same way to the use of tuning forks.

Reflex Points

In this section you are given two aspects to consider in sound or vibrational therapy. First, are the symptoms that occur in the body and secondly, reflexing the areas on the body to take care of the problems. You will be using tuning forks, which produce the proper sound in Hz to assist the body in healing. Lets say for the sake of argument that every part of our body resonates at a different frequency. A healthy body is in tune. The body is like a huge orchestra that is playing the grand symphony of your life. When everyone is in tune and playing at the same beat it works. If someone is having a bad day, or is thinking about something negative, or maybe playing out of tune, it doesn't work.

Every organ of our body has a frequency or a note playing at the same time. This creates harmonics that give us health. If the frequency is too low, a string is too loose. If the frequency is too high, it is to tight. Or the string can snap. No matter what it is you hear it is still out. With the body you can't hear what is out, however the body will produce SYMPTOMS to let you know something is out. In its own way it is telling you it needs to be tuned. The symptoms do not necessarily mean that's where or what the problem is. The whole body and everything in it are connected. If something is out somewhere a symptom may show up somewhere else. Which may be the place we should be working on rather then trying to take care of the symptom. How we do this is to reflex the place where the problem is. This means there is a place on the body to send a frequency to correct what is out. This brings it back into tune, like tapping your knee and your leg moves. You have reflexed the knee with a force and produced an action. The same holds true with tuning forks when reflexed to a point on the body. It will in turn cause an action on the rest of the body. To reflex the area or wash over it, simply point the prongs of the fork (after it is vibrating) at the area you are reflexing to. Listed below are symptoms that show up and where to reflex the sound; in other words, where to point the tuning fork.

C or Red Fork *Symptom:* poor circulation, iron deficiency anemia and blood disorders, paralysis, swollen ankles and cold feet, lumbago, stiff joints, constipation or diarrhea, sadness.
Reflex to: colon, neck, knees, nose

D or Orange Fork *Symptom:* asthma, bronchitis, gout, gallstones, obesity, purification and removal of toxins and poisons, lethargy and apathy
Reflex to: breasts, reproductive organs, perinea floor, feet and tongue
E or Yellow Fork *Symptom:* constipation, indigestion, flatulence, liver and gastrointestinal disorders, coughs, headache, poor skin condition, sluggishness, boredom

Reflex to: head, eyes, solar plexus, umbilical area, and thighs
F or Green Fork *Symptom:* hay fever, allergies, head colds, trauma and shock, colic, exhaustion, ulcers, sleeplessness, high blood pressure, irritability, back pain, dry skin
Reflex to: kidneys, shoulder, chest colon, suprarenal gland, calves, and ankles

G or Blue Fork *Symptom:* Laryngitis, tonsillitis and throat infections, headaches, eye problems, skin disorders and itching, vomiting, muscular spasms, menstruation pains, fevers
Reflex to: reproductive system, saliva, and hair

A or Purple Fork *Symptom:* nervous ailments, convulsions, obsessions, balance disorders, excessive bleeding, swelling and palsy, shingles
Reflex to: sacrum (base of spine)

B or Violet Fork *Symptom:* neuralgia, cramps and inflammatory pains, glandular imbalance, immune deficiency, processing vitamins, goiters, and nervous disorders
Reflex to: entire body

TUNING THE ORGANS

The Organ Tuning Forks

Just like a symphony orchestra, when the organs are all in balance and healthy they sing a harmonic song of wholeness. But when one or more organ is out of balance or diseased they create a dis-functoning system effecting the other organs. By using the Organ Tuning Fork Set one can retune the organs back into balance creating a synergistic healthy flow of life force energy. This chapter explains the process and procedure necessary to retune or rebalance the organs into a normal healthy function.

The set has 14 forks, one for each of the major organs and essential parts of the physical body. These forks are tuned to the frequencies of healthy human tissue. They can be used to elevate the body to a balanced state of health. They most efficient used in conjunction with the chakra forks in healing, but can also be used individually for a specific issue. To bring the body into alignment, balance the charkas first & then use the Organ Tuning Fork Set to correct the frequency of each organ.

The human body uses its organs to support it in staying balanced. For example if the lungs are not operating at the level of efficiency that they were meant to be, the oxygen to the rest of the body is lessened. From this the rest of the body does not have what it needs to operate correctly. When we can change the way an organ is functioning, we can get the body back into balance.

To assist you in retuning the organs find listed the organs and the fork(s) to use in the process. Tap the tuning fork to get it vibrating and place the stem on or over the organ until it stops vibrating. This will assist in releasing stagnant energy, which isn't serving the organ well. Then to put energy into the organ turn the fork the other way around so that the stem is facing away from the organ.

Another way to retune the organs is by applying the tuning forks to the reflex points on the bottom of the feet. This is great if there are some difficult areas to reach. The client doesn't need to undress for the processes - you can just have him/her remove shoes and socks.

The Organs Tuning Fork Set is considered an advance set, and can be used to balance certain organs or to clear a specific emotions or issues. Using a specific Organ tuning fork to clear a specific emotion or issue can be more direct and save time when used with other healing modalities. Find below a list of the organs & their corresponding note, frequency and relevant emotions or thoughts, which could create imbalance.

Blood - E 321.9 Hz. Lack of Joy.
Adrenals - B 492.8 Hz. Anxiety.
Kidneys - Eb 319.88 Hz. Fear, disappointment, failure.
Liver - Eb 317.83 Hz. Anger.
Bladder - F 352 Hz. Anxiety, fear of letting go.
Intestines - C# 281 Hz. Assimilation & absorption.
Lungs - A 220 Hz. Grief, depression, unworthy.
Colon - F 176 Hz. Releasing the past.
Gall Bladder - E 164.3 Hz. Pride, hard thoughts.
Pancreas - C# 117.3 Hz. Deep sorrow, a need to control.
Stomach - A 110 Hz. Fear of the new, dread.
Brain - Eb 315.8 Hz. Stubborn, fear, self criticism, refusing to change.
Muscles - E 324 Hz. Resistance to new experiences.

Adrenals Tuning Fork

This fork is to bring balance to the adrenals, and is tuned to the frequencies of a healthy adrenal gland. It can be used to elevate the adrenals to a balanced state of health. Strike the fork on a rubber hockey puck to get it vibrating then wave the fork over the area of the adrenals for 20 seconds. Repeat the process again for another 20 seconds.

Bladder Tuning Fork

This fork is to bring balance to the Bladder, and is tuned to the frequencies of a healthy Bladder. It can be used to elevate the bladder to a balanced state of health. Strike the fork on a rubber hockey puck, then wave the tuning fork over the Bladder area, this will bring the Bladder into balance.

Blood Tuning Fork

This fork is to bring balance to the blood system, and is tuned to the frequencies of a healthy blood system. It can be used to elevate the blood to a balanced state of health. Strike the fork on a rubber hockey puck, then while vibrating place the fork 8 inches above the heart area, waving the fork for 20 seconds. This will send the vibrational frequency into the blood stream creating a healthy flow of blood.

Brain Tuning Fork

The brain takes on external stimuli through the sensory system. Touch, taste, smell, sight and sound are all transmitted to the brain, however the connections that allow brain cells to process this information will become distorted if lacking the proper stimulation. Sensory deprivation has a significant impact on the brain.

Balancing the Sides of the Brain

Stand at the head of the healing table facing the person lying on the table face up. Tap the Brain fork to start it vibrating, then place the fork with the stem placed on the right side of the temple for 20 seconds. Then repeat the process on the left temple, for 20 seconds. Tap the fork again and move the fork to above the ears (in the small indentation), tap the fork again and do the other side (above the ear) for 20 seconds. Tap again and place the stem in the small indentation behind the ear lobe. Repeat to other ear. Next tap again and place the stem of the brain fork on the crown of the head. Then use the Om fork by placing the Om fork (when vibrating) 4 inches from the ear for 20 seconds, the repeat the process on the other ear. This will bring the brain organ back into a balanced frequency.

Colon Tuning Fork
This fork is to bring balance to the colon, and is tuned to the frequencies of healthy colon. It can be used to elevate the organ to a balanced state of health. Strike the fork on a rubber hockey puck, once the fork is vibrating wave the fork over the colon area for 20 seconds, this will bring the colon into harmonic balance.

Gall Bladder Tuning Fork
This fork is to bring balance to the Gall Bladder, and is tuned to the frequencies of a healthy Gall Bladder. It can be used to elevate the Gall Bladder to a balanced state of health. Strike the fork on a rubber hockey puck, once the fork is vibrating wave the fork over the Gall Bladder area for 20 seconds, this will bring the Gall Bladder into harmonic balance.

Intestines Tuning Fork
This fork is part of the Organ Tuning Forks Set. This fork is to bring balance to the Intestines, and is tuned to the frequencies of healthy Intestines. It can be used to elevate the Intestines to a balanced state of health. Strike the fork on a rubber hockey puck, once the fork is vibrating wave the fork over the Gall Bladder area for 20 seconds, this will bring the Gall Bladder into harmonic balance.

Kidneys Tuning Fork

This fork is to bring balance to the kidneys, and is tuned to the frequencies of healthy kidneys. It can be used to elevate the kidneys to a balanced state of health. Strike the tuning fork on a rubber hockey puck, once the tuning fork is vibrating wave the tuning fork over the Kidney area, this will bring the Kidney into balance.

Liver Tuning Fork
This fork is to bring balance to the liver, and is tuned to the frequencies of healthy liver tissue. It can be used to elevate the liver to a balanced state of health. Use the Liver tuning fork by striking the fork on a rubber hockey puck, once the tuning fork is vibrating, wave the tuning fork over the Liver area, this will bring the Liver into balance.

Lungs Tuning Fork
This fork is to bring balance to the Lungs, and is tuned to the frequencies of healthy Lungs. It can be used to elevate the Lungs to a balanced state of health. Use the Lung tuning forks by striking it on a rubber hockey puck, once the fork is vibrating wave the fork over the lungs over 20 seconds, this will bring the Lungs into balance.

Muscles Tuning Fork
This fork is to bring balance to the Muscles, and is tuned to the frequencies of healthy Muscles. It can be used to elevate the Muscles to a balanced state of health. Use the Muscles tuning fork by striking it on a rubber hockey puck, once the fork is vibrating wave the fork over the Muscles of the body (especially over muscles that are sore, strained or injured), this would bring the Muscles into balance.

Pancreas Tuning Fork
This fork is to bring balance to the Pancreas, and is tuned to the frequencies of a healthy Pancreas. It can be used to elevate the Pancreas to a balanced state of health.

Stomach Tuning Fork
This fork is to bring balance to the stomach, and is tuned to the frequencies of healthy stomach tissue. It can be used to elevate the stomach to a balanced state of health. Use the Stomach tuning fork by striking it on a rubber hockey puck, once the fork is vibrating wave the fork over the stomach area for 20 seconds, this will bring the Stomach into balance.

Body Tuning

Body Tuning is a phrase coined by John Beaulieu, N.D., author of "Music and Sound in the Healing Arts", that describes the use of tuning forks called Body Tuners. Body Tuning is a powerful way of using sound vibrations to resonate the body, brain, and etheric fields. The specific tuning forks used are a C fork of 256 Hz and a G fork of 384 Hz.

These two forks vibrate at a ratio of 2:3, which is considered sacred in many traditions that have an understanding of the relationship of mathematics to the universe. These two forks, when used in combination, produce a perfect fifth interval and are said to open a gateway for healing and higher consciousness. John Beaulieu, N.D., says that this fifth interval has many benefits such as counteracting depression, making joints more mobile, balancing the earth with the spirit, balancing the heart, pituitary gland, and sphenoid bone as well as balancing the sympathetic and parasympathetic nervous system.

When both forks are struck and brought to the ears the brain hears a third tone that brings the entire nervous system into balance and integrates the mind and body. Within 30 seconds it may be possible to reach a state of deep relaxation that might otherwise take you 45 minutes to achieve through meditation alone. They also balance both hemispheres of the brain, the auric field, and release energy blocks. The tones can alleviate depression, improve joint mobility, and balance the spirit with the earth. This method can also be used to prepare a client for any type of healing session including chakra balancing.

Procedure

Strike both forks and bring them to your ears or the ears of your client. You may strike the forks as often as is necessary to let them experience the tones and create a deep resonance within the head. Make sure to switch sides with the forks as you do this. You might also use the forks to wash over the body or sweep the energy field. Let your intuition guide you in this regard.

USING TUNING FORKS WITH REFLEXOLOGY

Tuning forks can also be use when giving a reflexology treatment. Using any reflexology chart you need only locate the desired reflexology point. Then, using a chakra chart that lists the body organs associated with each individual chakra, find the chakra that corresponds to the desired organ or body part.

From this it is easy to choose the appropriate tuning fork to be used. For example, if the reflexologist needed to work on the reflex point related to the spleen, they would use a chakra chart and note that the spleen was related to the Sacral chakra. The Sacral chakra corresponds to the "D" tuning fork. So the reflexologist would use the "D" tuning fork to work on the spleen reflex point. The tuning fork would be used by activating and placing the stem directly on the reflex point or allowing the vibrations to wash over the area.

In the case of reflexing a kidney point the reflexologist would choose two tuning forks, the "C" and the "D", since the kidneys are related to both the Root and the Sacral chakra. They could be used individually, one at a time, or together by striking them together carefully.

A List of Tuning Forks

The Ozone (O_3) Fork

O_3 is the symbol for ozone, three oxygen molecules bonded together. Ozone in the atmosphere keeps our planet and the life on it safe from the harmful effects of ultraviolet radiation. Ozone has other useful properties such as keeping the air inside our homes clean. Ozone purifiers remove harmful bacteria, viruses, dust, and other allergens from the air.

Ozone is an unstable molecule. To become stable it must lose one of its oxygen molecules and become O_2. The molecule thrown off attaches to viruses or bacteria and kills them. It also attaches to dust and allergens and removes them from the air we breathe.

Ozone has yet another very important benefit to humans. When abnormal cells are subjected to ozone they cannot reproduce more of themselves. When the abnormal cell, such as a cancer cell, is prevented from reproducing, our immune systems can then attack and destroy them.

Ozone can be produced by a thunderstorm, by man made devices, or by the human body. The ozone fork vibrates at a bit over 78 Hz, which is above the range needed to produce ozone in the body. The frequency of ozone in the body and the frequency of the tuning fork will resonate at the same frequency. This will enhance the production of ozone in the body wherever the fork is placed. The ozone fork can be washed over the body area or placed directly on the spot that needs treatment.

To Use

If an infection or virus is present point the tines at the infection and wash over the area as needed. You may also place the stem on any spot where there might be a virus problem allowing the vibration to enter the body.

For tumors, place the stem on the tumor. The vibrations will prohibit the growth of abnormal cells allowing the immune system to take over and destroy them. Keep in mind that with any medical problems you still need the advice and treatment of medical professionals.

The ozone fork is also used on any of the points that are used for viral or bacterial treatments in Acupuncture, Acupressure, or AcuTuning. It is available from Angel Gate Creations, www.teachonlylove.com.

The Nerve Fork

A nerve fires at a frequency of 50 Hz carrying a message from the brain or to the brain. When some trauma to the body occurs, the nerve tells the brain something is out. The brain reacts to this process by correcting it. If the damage is too great for the brain to repair easily, it starts sending endorphins to ease the pain. If the damage is to the nerve, the frequency for information is hindered in the flow to the brain.

This tuning fork can be used to relive pain from pulled or strained muscles. It is also excellent fork for removing those knots that develop in the muscles. It will help in releasing the tightness of cramps so that the muscle will relax and the brain will send the endorphins to help with the pain. Place the end of the stem on the area where there is pain. You may also place the side of the stem in the same area. On the weighted end of the tuning fork pinch the two ends together and slide your fingers off quickly. Hitting the end of the fork on a hard rubber object is not needed to cause the maximum amount of vibration.

For wounds and bruises DO NOT place the stem side of the tuning fork on the area. Instead pinch the end of the tuning fork and point that at the wound or bruise moving in a circular motion.

<u>Knots in the Muscle</u>

Place the stem point of the Nerve fork on the knot in the muscle. Pinch the end of the fork to make it vibrate. If this causes pain you may want to vibrate the fork and then roll the side of the stem over the spot first to loosen it up. REMEMBER you don't have to press hard to have the vibrations work on the muscle. Once you have sent the 50 Hz into the muscle you will want to place Michaels oil over the spot. Again use the 50 Hz fork by applying the point or the side of the stem. In no time at all you will feel the knot release.

Cramps

Place the side of the stem on the muscle and roll it back and forth over the area. This will help the muscle to relax. Michael's oil mixed with equal amounts of Shekinah oil will work wonders with calming the cramping muscle.

Shoulder Pain

From muscle strain of over working or too much typing the 50 Hz can be used by running the stem point over the area where it hurts. You should start to feel the endorphins being released along with the pain and stiffness subsiding.

Carpel Tunnel and Sciatica

Using the stem point, run it down the pain line slowly. You will have to vibrate the fork several times to sent the vibrations down the entire length of the pain line. Again you may want to use Michael's oil and the Shekinah oil.

Numbness

For numbness, take the stem and place it on the area. I have found that the oil of Gabriel works well in this process because of its gentleness and healing qualities. Constricted nerves should open rather easily, however, severely damaged nerves will take more time to repair themselves. In either case repeat the tuning process until feeling returns.

The Psychic Fork Set

The Psychic Fork Set is a set of 5 forks that are set to the brain waves of someone who is proficient in these gifts. Each of us possesses these gifts, even if we do not use them or are even aware of them. These frequencies are used to tune your brain to the frequencies of having these psychic gifts. Some have experiences immediately while others have to continue to practice and have patience. Be open to allowing yourself to come to these frequencies within your own being. The forks work very well with the CD set, because you have the best of both worlds - the meditating process and the actual vibrations being placed on the areas to be tuned.

Kundalini Brain Wave

The Kundalini tuning fork holds the same frequency as that of a Master passing this energy or the person receiving the experiencing of it. Kundalini can be thought of as a rich source of psychic or libidinous energy in our unconscious. This energy can be used to heighten the spiritual experience or the sexual experience and then again both. It is the energy of creation and it is this energy you tap into whenever you are manifesting anything. This tuning fork has been designed in its frequency to stimulate the flow of Kundalini energy.

INSTRUCTIONS:
The first thing you will need to do is center yourself; reach that place in meditation of allowance, where you let go of all judgments and just open yourself to receive. Pinch the weighted ends together and quickly slide your fingers away letting the prongs of the tuning fork vibrate. As the tuning fork vibrates place it on the base of the spine where it meets the skull. The point of the fork should be in the soft tissue just below the skull with the stem of the fork resting against the base of the skull. You may need to pinch the ends together several times to keep the vibration going to carry the frequency to the brain. For those of you that have received "shaktipat" before, you will notice how quickly the experience returns. For those of you that have not I can tell you this, Shakti is the equivalent to a combined physical and spiritual orgasm, without an ejaculation and can last hours.

Third Eye Brain Wave

This tuning fork is set to the brain waves of a fully functioning and focused third eye. This is designed to help those that have not been able to use their third eye to do so. As the brain waves are reproduced in the brain you will be able to start training your third eye to see clearly. Colors will become more rich and vibrant and you will be able to see energies from things with your eyes closed. As you become proficient in third eye work with your eyes closed, you will reach a point where you can see auras with your eyes open. You will be able to look into a body and see things that are out in the way of diseases.

INSTRUCTIONS:
The first thing you will need to do is center yourself, reach that place in meditation of allowance, where you let go of all judgments and just open yourself to receive. Pinch the weighted ends together and quickly slide your fingers away letting the prongs of the tuning fork vibrate. Place the tuning fork just above the third eye, which is located in the center of your forehead. Close your physical eyes and notice what you see. Most people see black; so don't get discouraged if that is what you see. Bring to mind a color, preferably a sky blue emanating in the area of the third eye. As you begin to see this color you will notice it begins to fill all that you are seeing. You may have to vibrate the tuning fork several times as the vibration lessens. When you can see a sky blue color you are now ready to bring to mind other colors. After you master the colors, you can start focusing on different objects and people with your third eye. When that is mastered and you can use your third eye to see color and objects, you are well on your way to seeing auras. Continue to practice until you become proficient at seeing auras and then you can begin to look inside bodies for things that are out.

Total Knowing Brain Wave

Total knowing comes from another realm of awareness. This tuning fork is designed to get you to that realm of knowing. Most people operate in only two realms of knowing. The first realm is "I know I know". This is very helpful to us as it is from this knowing we go about our lives. We do the work we know how to do. We run a family in the way we know works. We do the same with choosing our friends or buying the things we need in our lives to be happy. The second realm is "I know I don't know". This is helpful in our lives, because if we know we don't know; we can learn. We can get the education we need to get the promotion at work. We can learn better ways to participate with our families where everyone feels loved and empowered. When we read instructions to fix or put something together we are operation in this realm.

The third realm is "I don't know I don't know". This is the realm of self- discovery that is very helpful in the growth process of a person. As teenagers we are all geniuses that can't understand how our mother and father ever made it this far being as stupid as they are. We know all there is to know or think we do. When we mature in life we begin to know that there are many thing we didn't know we didn't know.

The fourth realm is " I don't know I know". This happens when we have an epiphany or what is called an "A Ha" moment. These are not the times when we read it or someone told us what to think. Oh, no. These are the times when we are able to reach into the brain wave patterns that allow us to draw on total knowing. Not as an understanding of it but a natural knowing of a universal truth.

INSTRUCTIONS:

The first thing you will need to do is center yourself; reach that place in meditation of allowance, where you let go of all judgments and just open yourself to receive. Pinch the weighted ends together and quickly slide your fingers away letting the prongs of the tuning fork vibrate. For this tuning you will need to alternate from one side of the forehead to the other beginning with the left side. Place the point or the stem of the fork along the hairline in the corners of the forehead, directly above the temples. We are activating the brain wave in the frontal lobes. As these brain waves change and the brain begins to become accustom to operating at this frequency you will start having A Ha's. Things that have not been working in your life for sometime will start opening up to you. There will be solutions to problems that you never thought of before profoundly changing the way you think about life and you in it.

P.S.I. Brain Wave

This psychic tuning fork is designed to raise your level of psychic ability. The brain waves are set to enhance your perception far beyond just a good guess. When you can train your brain to use these waves you will be able to use the psychic gifts that are innate in all of us. It has been said we only use 10% of our brains true power. This 10% has nothing to do with how smart someone is. This has everything to do with how much of the gray matter is operating at any given time. The more of the brain that is being used the more we are aware of The more we can tap into the better we are in having the happy lives we want.

INSTRUCTIONS:
The first thing you will need to do is center yourself; reach that place in meditation of allowance, where you let go of all judgments and just open yourself to receive. Pinch the weighted ends together and quickly slide your fingers away letting the prongs of the tuning fork vibrate. For this tuning you will need to alternate from one side of the forehead to the other, beginning with the left side. Place the point or the stem of the fork along the hairline in the corners of the forehead, directly above the temples. We are activating the brain waves in the frontal lobes. As you tune your brain to these frequencies the more you will be able to pick up when working with other people. The more you will be able to pick up in your life and what is going on around you. Your ability to avoid situations that could lead to trouble will increase vastly along with you being able to take advantage of situations for your benefit. Lastly as you reach the place where you master the use of these brain waves there comes the ability to move objects.

Change Matter Brain Waves

This tuning fork is designed to take the brain waves to a much higher level. It is from these brain waves that very few people can alter mater. There is a catch with these brain waves. Which is simply this, unless you have mastered the lower frequencies and can come into these brain waves with a complete benevolent and loving body, mind, and soul combined you will not be able to change matter. The good news is if you can master the lower levels to get you to this point you will be in that place of love.

INSTRUCTIONS:
The first thing you will need to do is center yourself; reach that place in meditation of allowance, where you let go of all judgments and just open yourself to receive. Pinch the weighted ends together and quickly slide your fingers away letting the prongs of the tuning fork vibrate. For this tuning you will need to alternate from one side of the forehead to the other, beginning with the left side. Place the point or the stem of the fork along the hairline in the corners of the forehead, directly above the temples. We are activating the brain waves in the frontal lobes. You will know when you get there.

Transmutation Brain Wave
Creation or Creation 2

This tuning fork is the frequency of the very structure of the DNA vibration. We call it the Creation fork (sold separately from the set). Scientists are using this frequency to rejuvenate and repair DNA. What they have been able to accomplish with it is nothing to what you can do if you can tune your brain waves to this frequency.

INSTRUCTIONS:
The first thing you will need to do is center yourself; reach that place in meditation of allowance, where you let go of all judgments and just open yourself to receive. The Creation tuning fork is either weighted or not, so you will need to tap the prongs on something made of hard rubber to get it vibrating or pinch the prongs together if weighted. For this tuning you will need to alternate from one side of the forehead to the other, beginning with the left side. Place the point or the stem of the fork along the hairline in the corners of the forehead, directly above the temples. We are activating the brain waves in the frontal lobes. You will know when you get there.

Astral/Mental Projection Wave

This tuning fork (not included in the set) is the frequency of conscious thoughts. These are the thoughts you are aware of having or that you intentionally put your mind too. This makes this frequency great for improving your ability to communicate with others. You can focus on mentally projecting your thoughts to another so they understand what it is that you are saying. For the most part we do not think in words but pictures. It can also be used to astrally project your Higher Self for travel in the astral realm for self-discovery and learning.

INSTRUCTIONS:

The first thing you will need to do is center yourself; reach that place in meditation of allowance, where you let go of all judgments and just open yourself to receive. The Astral/Mental tuning fork is weighted so pinch the prongs together to get it vibrating. For this tuning you will need to place the fork on the crown and then both of the temples, alternate from one side of the forehead to the other. We are activating the brain waves in the frontal lobes. You will know when you get there.

Standard Chakra Set

Tuned to the vibrations of the chakras. The handles are color coded to make them easier to use in chakra alignments and Crystaline reiki sessions

Tree of Life Tuning Forks

This awesome set includes the Sacred Solfeggio scale. They are used in conjunction with the chakra forks in healing. This set includes 11 forks, each imprinted with the angels' names and color coded for easy identification. Each fork has a different use in healing from correcting DNA to rejuvenating cells.

Sefirot Tuning Forks

The Sefirot tuning forks are a set of 11 forks that are used for attuning the angelic forks in the Tree of Life set. Each Sefirot has a frequency with a numerical value that equals three, six or nine the same as the Tree of Life set.

Creation Frequency

This fork is combined with the others to cause things to happen or to create things. It can be used alone or with the Gabriel fork to repair damaged portions of DNA. It can also be used alone or with the Shekinah fork to destroy cancer cells. It also will move bones and joints back into place when they are out of alignment. It will also repair and rebuild muscles and tissue. These are just a few of the amazing things we are discovering about this frequency the possibilities are endless.

Circulation Fork

The frequency of the Circulation fork is used to stimulate the flow of blood to areas of the body. Arthritis is a prime example of poor circulation in the joints. Once the flow of blood is returned to the damaged areas it will start to heal its self. The Circulation forks frequency works on Diabetes and other diseases, as well.

To use the Circulation fork simply start it vibrating by tapping it on the heal of the hand. Once it is vibrating place the tip of the stem/handle on the joint or area where there is stiffness or pain. Allow the tuning fork tip to remain on the area until it stops vibrating and then repeat the process three to four more times. Massaging or vigorously rubbing the area helps to spread the frequency vibration especially applying Michael's oil when massaging the area.

With diabetes you will want to cover as much area as possible. The process is the same for vibrating the fork and placement. However, you will need to work in areas about 10 inches apart. Pick an area where you want to stimulate blood flow and place the stem tip on there. Let the fork vibrate until it stops. Do this 3 to 4 times before moving on to another area. You may then massage the area you just worked on or massage all of the areas when you have finished with the fork. You may do this process several times during the day for faster results but it is not necessary. Once a week will help in restoring the flow of blood to the areas but it will take longer to have the desired results.

This frequency has also been found to reduce cholesterol. Simply start the fork vibrating and place over the area of the liver.

Psychic Set

The psychic set of tuning forks can be used to enhance one's intuitive and psychic abilities, those forks consists of the PSI fork, at 252.20 hertz, the change matter fork at 351.20 hertz, the total knowing fork at 108.40 herta, the third eye fork at 82.80 hertz and the Kundalini fork at 55.60 hertz. Using these specific forks, after balancing the chakras can stimulate the individual into experiencing a state of enhanced psychic abilities, which can be come permeate if used over a specific time frame in the manner layout in the Psychic set manual.

Afterthoughts- 2023

The healing art of sound healing with tuning forks has gone through a lot of changes, research and expansion since I start working as a certified Tuning Fork Practitioner in 2001.I still use tuning forks in my healing practice, and teach the art of tuning fork healing and how to use it with other modalities, such as massage, Reiki. Crystal and Gemstone Healing, Intuitive Healing,and Spititual Healing.

 I have even worked with Chiropractors who have used tuning forks in their healing practice, as well as Acupuncturists who have used them in their healing practice. Tuning forks are part of Vibrational Medicine and will hopefully be embraced by holistic healthcare providers as well as mainstream medical care providers, to provide for the best care for their clients/patients.

As people become aware of how to utilize tuning forks in their own self care, we will all become healthier and more balanced in our journey called life.

The future holds promising research possibilities for tuning forks and their use in the healing of people and animals.

If you enjoy this book, perhaps you will enjoy reading some of my other books as well:

Quantum Healing: The synergy of Chiropractic and Reiki, co-authored with Dr. Pat Doughtery,D.C.

Advanced Sound Healing with Tuning Forks

Atlantean Reiki: Healing Knowledge from a lost civilization

Crystal Reiki Workbook

Crystaline Reiki: A New Frequency of Healing

Crystal & Gemstone Healing: Using Using Crystals and Gemstones in the art of Healing

Medical Intuition Handbook: An Overview of Medical Intuition, its history and famous Medical :Intuitive's of the World

Vibrational Yoga: Using Voice Sounds in the Yogic Experience

Upcoming Books:
                By Charles Lightwalker

Medical Intuition and Muscle Testing Co-Authored with Dr. Pat Doughtery

Life Changing Lesson from an Elder: Learning the Metis Medicine Ways Co-Authored with Charles Edwards, Ph.D.

Musings: A collection of Poetry, Writings & Thoughts

Bits and Pieces :A collection of philosophy according to Charles Lightwalker

Learning to Channel Workbook

Charles is a member of the following professional organizations:

- International Association of Medical Intuitives
- Natural Healers Association
- International Holistic Therapies Directory
- Natural Health Resource Alliance
- Spiritual Healers and Earth Stewards
- The Metaphysical Research Society
- Alternative Healthcare Alliance/Spokane
- Sound Healers Of Washington
- International Association of Healthcare Practitioners
- American Holistic Health Association
- Sound Healer Association
- World Reiki Association
- International Association of Sound healers
- Society for Shamanic Practitioners
- National Federation of Spiritual Healers (U.K.)

THE HISTORY OF SOUND HEALING AND THE USE OF TUNING FORKS IN THERAPUTIC SOUND HEALING

By Charles Lightwalker

In 1550 in Pavia, Italy, Girolamo Cardano, a physician, mathematician and astrologer, noticed how sound was being perceived through the skin. In 1553 in Padua, Italy, H. Capivacci, a physician, noticed that this knowledge of sound being perceived through the skin might be used as a diagnostic tool for differentiating between hearing disorders located in the middle ear or in the acoustic nerve. In 1684, German physician G. C. Schelhammer tried using a common cutlery fork to enhance the experiments that Cardano and Capivacci were working on. In 1711 in England, Royal trumpeter and luteist, John Shore, created the first tuning fork. At that time, he lovingly and jokingly called it a pitch fork. It was made of steel and had a pitch of A423.5. In 1800, German physicist E.F.F. Chladni, along with others, constructed a complete musical instrument based on sets of tuning forks. In 1834, J.H. Scheibler presented a set of 54 tuning forks covering ranges from 220 Hz to 440Hz. Later, in Paris, J. Lissajous constructed a tuning fork with a resonance box. Also in Paris, German physicist K. R. Koening invented a tuning fork, which was kept in continuous vibration by a clockwork. In 1863 in Heidelberg, physiologist H. Helmholtz, used sets of electromagnetically powered tuning forks for his experiments on the sensations of tone. Tuning forks were indispensible instruments for producing defined sinusoidal vibrations and used as a diagnostic tool in otology. The most common system of determining the pitch of all twelve notes in a octave is the Equal temperament. The standard pitch here is A440. As a side note, equal temperament was proposed by Aristoxenus, a pupil of Aristotle, and had been in use in China for some centuries. Mr. Hipkins, the head piano tuner in 1846, was instructed by

Walter Broadwood to instruct his piano tuners in the use of equal temperament. To do this, he used two tuning forks; one for meantone at A433.5 and one for equal temperament at A436. Even though musicians were among the first people to work with pitch, scientist enjoyed sharing knowledge and use of the tuning fork also. As far back as 583 BC, when the Greek philosopher, Pythagorus, made a device called the monochord and set the pitch to 256Hz.. The Egyptians and Greeks used the monochord to make intricate mathematical calculations. It wasn't until around 1834 when a group of German physicists was able to use a mechanical stroboscopic device, that they were able to determine that the pitch of the tuning fork was at A440cps (which later was expressed as A440Hz). Even though the pitch of the note "A" in the 17th century varied from 373.3 Hz to 402.0 Hz, on July 27, 1987, the International society of Piano Builders and Technicians unanimously support A=440 Hz. as the international pitch standard for piano manufacturers and for modern piano and orchestral tuning.

Who Uses Tuning Forks in Sound Healing

By *Charles Lightwalker*

Everyday people and practitioners in the Healing Arts are using tuning forks to positively alter the body's biochemistry. Sound enhances the healing effects of all energy therapy practices.

People who use tuning forks are often involved with:

- Acupuncturists
- Chiropractors
- Polarity Therapy
- Crystaline Reiki Therapy
- Massage Therapy
- Yoga Therapy
- Hypnotherapy
- Psychotherapy
- Meditation
- Reflexology
- Shamanic Healing

And anyone interested in alternative healing modalities and pain management. You can use tuning forks and sound to experience deep levels of healing by bringing your body back to its fundamental pulse and by connecting you to your Core Rhythm.

Why are so many people using Tuning Forks?

- Provides instantaneous, deep state of relaxation
- Improves mental clarity and brain functioning
- Increases your level of physical energy and mental concentration (Energy Fork)
- Relieves stress by drawing your body into a centered space

- Enhances massage, acupressure, dream-work and meditation
- Brings your nervous system into balance (Nerve fork)
- Integrates left and right brain thought patterns
- Increase psychic abilities (Psychic Set)

When you tap the tuning forks, you awaken the life energy of your cells and start them puffing, creating a centered, happy feeling inside. Align your body and mind with the world's best sound healing technologies.

With tuning forks you'll be able to:

- Achieve deep relaxation and mind/body balance in seconds--not hours
- Reduce stress and muscular tension, spasms and pain nearly instantaneously (Nerve Fork)
- Increase blood flow and circulation by releasing constriction around targeted organs (Circulation fork)
- Transcend to higher levels of consciousness and access spiritual insights (Creation Fork)

Each tuning fork is calibrated at a specific frequency to address different areas of healing and development.

Six Sound Healing Facts to Consider
By Charles Lightwalker

Sound healing with tuning forks can be combined with other complimentary care healing modalities, such as chiropratic, crystal and Gemstone healing, massage therapy, Reiki healing, Shamanic healing, and yoga to enhance overall balance and healing for the client.

Here is six facts to consider about Sound Healing.

*Instruments: Various instruments like tuning forks, crystal bowls, Tibetan singing bowls, gongs, and even the human voice can be used in sound healing.

*Frequency Matters: Different sound frequencies interact differently with the body's energy (auric) fields.

*Binaural Beats: Binaural beats are a type of sound wave therapy that uses different frequencies tones in each ear, which are then processed by the brain into a single beat. This healing method said to induce states of relaxation, focus, or creativity depending on the frequency used.

*Brainwave Entrainment: Brainwave entrainment involves synchronizing brain wave frequencies to specific rhythms. This has been used to alter mental states, improve focus, or promote relaxation.

*Chakra Alignment: There are twelve Chakras-Energy Centers, each resonating with a specific frequency. Tuning Fork Practitioner use specific scientificllu calibrated tuning forks to balance these energy centers promoting physical, emotional, mental well being.

*Stess Reduction: Sound healing can promote deep states of relaxation and stress reduction.

List of Sound Healing
Tuning Fork Books References

Advanced Sound Healing with Tuning Forks, C.Lightwalker

Healing Sounds, J. Goldman

Stem Cells, Dr. Joe Crain

Acutuning 1,& 2, Dr. Joe Crain

Tuning Fork Therapy F. Milford

Opening the Psychic Pathways, C. Lightwalker

The Healing Power of Sound, M. Gaynor,M.D.

The Cosmic Octave, Hans Cousto

This by no means a complete list of excellent books on Sound healing. More books are listed in my advanced book.

www.ingramcontent.com/pod-product-compliance
Ingram Content Group UK Ltd.
Pitfield, Milton Keynes, MK11 3LW, UK
UKHW041421180426
11947UKWH00007B/228